The INVISIBLE Diet

BY: WILLIAM FARABAUGH

ISBN 0-7414-2510-6

Published by:

INFINITY
PUBLISHING.COM

1094 New DeHaven Street, Suite 100
West Conshohocken, PA 19428-2713
Info@buybooksontheweb.com
www.buybooksontheweb.com
Toll-free (877) BUY BOOK
Local Phone (610) 941-9999
Fax (610) 941-9959

Printed in the United States of America

Printed on Recycled Paper

Published July 2005

This book is dedicated to

My lovely wife,

My two wonderful children,

And

My mother and father

CONTENTS

PHASE 2: UNDERSTAND YOUR INNER-SELF AND UNLEASH THE THE POWER FROM WITHIN

PHASE 3: LOOK AT THINGS A LITTLE DIFFERENTLY AND APPLY YOUR KNOWLEDGE

CONTENTS

ACKNOWLEDGMENT

I must express my deepest appreciation to my wife, Debra, and my children, Erica and Luke, for their patience, kindness and understanding while pursuing my obsession. For pushing me on when all seemed so bleak. For your encouragement and your love. For your suggestions, criticism and input. You truly are responsible for this finished product.

Mom and dad, Dorothy and Earl, for always being there when I needed you most. Thank you for your love, support and suggestions.

Michelle Parsons, your suggestions helped me to believe in myself.

To all my family and friends that encouraged me in this venture. You know who you are.

Napoleon Hill, your inspirational book provided a catalyst for seeking a deeper understanding of the invisible forces that influence our lives.

PREFACE

PREFACE

Laid forth in this volume is a method/discipline to lose weight the "*EFFORTLESS WAY.*"

When I say effortless, I mean:

- No calorie counting
- No complicated exercises
- No special recipes
- No avoidance techniques
- No this, no that

This diet is as easy as walking down hill, swimming with the current, or having your back to the wind.

It is not my place to preach about WHAT to eat, HOW much to eat, WHERE to eat, or even WHEN to eat. That also goes for exercise. I will leave that to my knowledgeable compatriots who specialize in those subjects.

I am here to help you simplify your life with an all new way to achieve your ideal body weight. This is more of a "*mind over matter approach.*"

Most people view new diets with suspicion, and for good reason. Think about it, the first three letters in diet are **DIE.**

PREFACE

When you propose to take on a new diet, in most cases, you are preparing to: A) give something up, B) take on something new, or C) give up something and take on something new.

Unless you have been holed up under a rock or are less than mentally competent, you are aware of what is good and conversely, what is bad for you.

Most likely you have more of a **WAIT** problem, than a problem with your **WEIGHT**.

What I am saying is this; you already know what to do, and what not to do. You simply are reluctant to take action!

The Invisible Diet is designed to inspire action by providing you with a means to achieve effective weight loss in a meaningful, simplistic and lasting way. When you grasp the principles of this book, you will become master of your fate.

APPLICATION

USE ***THE INVISIBLE DIET*** TO:

- ACHIEVE WEIGHT LOSS
- INSPIRE OTHERS
- MOTIVATE YOURSELF AND OTHERS
- BECOME MORE PASSIONATE
- LIVE A MORE FULFILLING LIFE
- ELIMINATE PROCRASTINATION

PHASE 1

EVERYTHING HAPPENS FOR A REASON

INTRODUCTION

THINGS ARE ALWAYS AT THEIR BEST IN THEIR BEGINNING.

Blaise Pascal (1623-1662)

INTRO

The Invisible Diet exists due to my wife's "*practical*" request to lose weight, without altering her existing diet or exercise regime.

Simply put, she wanted to lose weight, and not suffer the discomfort of change!

Right! How practical is that, asking for something and giving nothing in return?

You and I have reasons to lose weight, and my wife's reason was to look and feel better. Also, her clothes fit a bit tight which bothered her.

My wife is a busy person. She works a full time job, exercises daily, eats what I consider to be a healthy diet, walks the dog regularly, and follows our children's sports schedule religiously. Whatever time she has left over, which is miniscule, is divided between family, hobbies and friends.

Yet, she wanted to lose five to ten pounds!

Here is where I get involved. Over the past few years I have devoted a significant portion of time studying personal fulfillment literature, and writings on the workings of the subconscious mind.

THE INVISIBLE DIET

My objective was to find, and develop, a systematic approach to obtain things that I considered previously unattainable.

Lo and behold, my wife's request fit the bill.

So the challenge began!

By applying what I had studied over the years, I was able to devise a weight loss system that fit my wife's needs.

The only thing missing was **belief**, belief that **this** weight loss system worked. My wife and I needed proof!

Before I presented the system to my wife, I decided to be the test subject.

I gave myself three months to lose fifteen pounds.

Three months later, I had shed a fraction over fifteen pounds using the system I developed.

VOILÀ

Armed with a system and results, I presented them to my wife.

INTRO

Keeping clear from my wife, I let her set confidential goals. All I asked her for were the results at the appropriate time.

FAST FORWARD

My wife looked me in the eye with a sense of disappointment. She had weighed herself and had only reached half of her goal.

What was your goal, I asked? She replied, "*ten pounds.*"

My wife had lost five pounds by doing **NO** additional exercise or messing with her life style! This had never happened to her before.

I was ecstatic about her results! By reaching half of the goal I felt I was on to something. Now I needed to know what she did to reach half the goal.

After questioning my wife about her adherence to the system I found, in short order, that she had not fully followed my instructions. Nor was she consistent in her application.

THE INVISIBLE DIET

Even with a partial application of the system, my wife was able to lose significant weight without changing her life style.

Where did the weight go? My wife and I both said the same thing when all was said and done. **The weight simply disappeared**. We did not recollect taking any specific action that would have influenced the results.

The weight did not "*simply disappear*", it gradually melted away due to small, nearly unrecognizable changes in our daily habits.

Your weight loss is predicated upon the compound effect of subtle changes.

LOGIC
VS.
EMOTION

WE KNOW THE GOOD, WE APPREHEND IT CLEARLY, BUT WE CAN'T BRING IT TO ACHIEVEMENT

Hippolytus (428 B.C.)

LOGIC vs. EMOTION

THE IMAGINARY BATTLEFIELD...

Logically, you and I should have no weight problem, or problems losing weight. There are so many sources of information available for the person choosing to lose weight that are time tested and proven. The problem is, we are not emotionally prepared to take action.

Because you and I are emotional beings, rather than logical ones (like Spock in the Star Trek series), we are more likely to experience the yo-yo effect of gaining and losing weight; rather than losing weight and keeping it off.

Let me give you an example:

Logic says, keep away from or be prudent in your consumption of fast food, alcohol, smokes, snack foods, etc. By employing logic, you are making conscious decisions.

You observe on the nightly news, read in the newspapers, and hear on the radio that Americans, in general, are significantly overweight.

There are plenty of statistics proclaiming the obvious---Americans are overweight. Do you need statistics to come to that conclusion? Just open your eyes and look about!

This problem is nothing short of an epidemic in nature. Surprisingly, the majority of those who are overweight appear to have resigned themselves to their plight.

You and I must individually address our shortcomings and take action before it is too late!

Once you recognize your overweight condition, you must take action. Who likes to get that shot in the arm to get rid of an illness? As severe as the overweight condition is, I am going to make the antidote for losing weight as painless as possible.

By understanding how the mind works, and by applying the principles of this book, you are able to influence the results of this and any diet in a favorable way.

Like a coin, your mind has two sides or spheres of influence which are:

A) conscious, logical side

B) subconscious, emotional side

The subconscious mind is also the seat of your imagination.

Of the two sides, the **subconscious** is the dominant force.

Let me give you an example:

Could you walk a mile on a smooth sandy beach overlooking a vast ocean on a calm pleasant day? Surely, you and the great majority of people could imagine doing that without hesitation, given enough time.

Now, introduce a hurricane, who could imagine walking the distance on this beach even with the incentive of great wealth? Just standing on the beach during the raging storm would be unimaginable for most people.

Obviously someone would try if given enough incentive.

What has really changed?

- Your perception has changed

What determines whether you take action or not?

- Your imagination.

The perceptions you develop are a function of the imagination which is a function of your subconscious mind.

I suggest what you ***IMAGINED*** changed! In the first case you imagined you could walk the beach. In the second case you imagined you could not. The beach did not change, only what you imagined would happen if you tried to walk the distance. When you imagine you cannot, your body obliges by stopping you.

Would you weather the storm and walk the distance if your life or the life of someone important to you depended upon it? That is a question only you can answer.

When you are overweight, your life certainly depends upon taking action.

Everyone knows that the quality of their life, their life span, health and the like are directly influenced by their weight.

LOGIC vs. EMOTION

The question is: Why have you not taken action up to now, or why have the actions that you have taken not worked?

Ultimately, the **actions** that lead to your weight loss, or your **lack of action** thereof, are directly influenced by your imagination or subconscious mind.

Prepare to lose weight, and keep it off, the "*effortless way*" by employing ***The Invisible Diet*** to influence your **subconscious imagination**.

THIS IS MY CONTRIBUTION

I LIVE IT

I LOVE IT

AND

I WANT TO SHARE IT WITH YOU!

CHANGE

GOD, GIVE US THE GRACE TO ACCEPT WITH SERENITY THE THINGS THAT CANNOT BE CHANGED, COURAGE TO CHANGE THE THINGS WHICH SHOULD BE CHANGED, AND THE WISDOM TO DISTINGUISH THE ONE FROM THE OTHER.

Reinhold Niebuhr (1892-1971)
The Serenity Prayer (1934)

CHANGE

BE NOT COMPLACENT...

This book is ultimately about change, how to create change by inspiring you to take action that leads to weight loss. I call this *will* to change *"desire"*, and desire is a call to action. This section addresses several methods to foster change.

You are unlikely to seek change until you see things from a different perspective. There is an old saying *"you cannot see the forest for the trees."* Rise above your problems, climb the mountain and look down upon the spectacle (your life).

Once you see your weight problem in the proper light, the remedy you seek becomes clear, and the actions you must take become evident.

When you genuinely desire change, you must do something different. If you keep on doing the same thing, you get the same results and nothing really changes.

I tell my children that they are "*hitting a wall*" when they experience **problems** getting something they desire. I suggest that they **look at**

things differently. Finding a way around the wall, jump over it, dig under it, knock it down, etc. In other words, do something (act), do not just focus on the problem (procrastinate); search for answers.

When you want something greatly, and encounter resistance, you must change your approach until you obtain that which you desire.

Creating desire is an answer to your weight problem.

By creating a strong enough desire, or *"will"* to change, you produce the necessary action to achieve your ideal body weight. The strongest form of desire you can develop is **obsession**.

When you repetitively say that you intend to achieve your ideal body weight, you develop an obsession within yourself that attainment of this goal is a must and that you are able to do it.

In preparation to lose weight and to achieve your ideal body weight, say to yourself: "*I intend to lose weight*." Say and think this often. When you repeat this enough, you become convinced that you must lose weight.

CHANGE

To elevate your desire to the level of obsession you must employ the principle of **autosuggestion** which is fully described in the section on **BELIEF.**

Obstacles crumble and fall by the wayside when you develop obsession.

"Wishing" is the shallowest form of desire. Wishing all day long gets you nowhere.

There is an Arabian proverb that goes like this: "W*ishing does not make a poor man rich*." You do not lose weight by just wishing to do so.

You are likely to change when you are not happy with your current body weight.

When you are **complacent** or **comfortable,** there is no need for change. You must want to change, desire change, and demand change for anything significant to occur in your life.

Accomplish this by saying to yourself ***"I do not accept this overweight condition any longer***!" Repeat this phrase often. This is a good way to get out of the comfort zone.

THE INVISIBLE DIET

When you feel resigned to a certain thing, like your current weight, there is no reason to change. You believe there is nothing you can do, therefore you do nothing. This is a trap.

This trap is constructed by a series of excuses that you created to justify your overweight condition. Excuses like:

- I do not have the time!
- I am too old!
- This is the way I should look at this age!

And the ultimate justification of all:

- It is healthy to be overweight!

Provide a convenient justification not to take action.

The way to dismantle this intricate trap is to take responsibility for your current weight. Do not let the past determine your future. Take action today! Analyze your excuses and dismantle them one by one.

CHANGE

Whenever I feel too old to do something, I remember a conversation with an elderly person, years ago, that had a profound effect on me. This gentleman basically said: "*These are the good old days; today IS the good old days. Take each day as it comes and make the best of it. This way, when you are old and in a nursing home, you will have no regrets.*"

To lose weight you must:

- **Convince** yourself that you are not happy with your current weight.

- **Believe** there is a way to lose weight that is compatible with your life style.

- **Believe you are capable** of bringing about the change necessary to achieve your ideal body weight.

- **Be willing** to do so.

Developing a "*willingness*" to change is a must. Do this by convincing yourself that you are not happy with your current weight. Make the attainment of your ideal body weight most important.

THE INVISIBLE DIET

To convince yourself that you are not happy with your current weight, you must have enough reasons "*why*" losing weight is important to you. The reasons must be numerous and have emotional weight, and then you will feel strongly about them.

Your "*willingness*" to lose weight multiplies, as the reasons for losing weight outnumber your reasons for not losing weight.

Now compile your own list of the "WHY'S", the reasons why you need to lose weight. Do this right here and now. Make it expansive. Give it importance.

CHANGE

REASONS WHY I MUST LOSE WEIGHT NOW!

(List them)

Imagine, in your minds eye, each reason to lose weight as a brick being piled on you. As the reasons accumulate you are being crushed by the weight. At a certain point, you must take action to relieve yourself of the pressure.

Change occurs primarily because you are willing to do so, and many times that willingness to change develops because your current condition is too painful, or there is too much pressure placed upon you.

The creation of pressure within you can be valuable when applied properly. Think of nearly worthless carbon buried deep within the Earth. With time, heat and pressure, the carbon can become a diamond.

The nearly worthless thought, *"I want to lose weight" is* formed into something of value, your ideal body weight, when you create enough pressure.

It is the pressure you create within yourself, the reasons **why** you must lose weight, that lead to the actions you take that eventually result in weight loss.

CHANGE

Think of your overweight condition as a tooth ache. The longer you decide to remedy the problem, the worse the problem gets. Finally, in desperation, you are driven to a remedy out of pain.

Tooth ache or not, you are driven to action, or lack thereof, by the forces of pleasure and pain. Let me explain.

Up to this point you enjoyed the pleasure of **inaction** because **action** represented pain in the form of:

- ❖ **DISAPPOINTMENT** (Previous efforts failed to produce the desired results therefore; since I have failed in the past I prefer not to repeat my mistakes. Why waste my time?)
- ❖ **SACRIFICE** (You have to give up something that you dearly enjoy.)
- ❖ **CHANGE** (You do not want to introduce an unknown into your life.)

What you need to do to avoid inaction is

represent action as pleasurable. Make the actions that you must take, in order to achieve your ideal body weight, appear easy, something to look forward to.

Your desire to lose weight must be coupled with a compatible weight loss program or system; otherwise conflict occurs in the form of inaction.

(This is a cautionary note. Selling illicit drugs is illegal. I do not sell drugs, buy them, consume them or finance the trade in them. The following is strictly an example for illustrative purposes.)

Take this premise; you need money. I could lay out, for you, a flawless plan to make a fortune by selling illegal drugs. Furthermore, I would finance the venture. Even though you may need the money in a big way, your decision to accept or deny this shady deal would rest on your deepest beliefs.

Now, let us say you believe illegal drugs are the root of all evil. Most likely you would turn-down the deal even though I may try to persuade you otherwise.

CHANGE

In the case above, the conflict rages between the need for money, and not wanting to do evil.

The solution is to find a compatible plan to make money in a legitimate way.

This rings true for your diet. Find a compatible solution to your diet problem and half the battle is won. The other half resides in believing in a system and then taking consistent action. If you do not believe in a specific diet or system, then it will not work for you, even though those who promote them may try to convince you otherwise.

Have you ever heard of Hakim's Razor? This basically says "*with all things being equal, the simplest explanation/answer is usually the right one*." So if this is true, wouldn't it be best to find and use the easiest diet possible?

Let's keep this simple.

Remember, by reducing or eliminating conflict and instilling compatibility you are more likely to reach your weight loss goal.

First, start by identifying and reducing conflict in your proposed diet.

THE INVISIBLE DIET

- ❖ You and I are busy people; therefore time must be kept to a minimum.
- ❖ Reduce your effort; you and I have plenty to do already.
- ❖ Dietary constraints must be nominal; who likes to be told what to eat anyway.

Now, let us create a compatible diet for you.

One that:

- ❖ Requires little or no time.
- ❖ Is effortless.
- ❖ Has no dietary constraint.

Wow, this sounds very much like ***The Invisible Diet!***

You are likely to embrace change when that change can yield great benefits with little to no physical effort.

You lose weight when the achievement of your ideal body weight becomes an obsession; something that you should have done yesterday.

CHANGE

Become enthusiastic about the achievement of your ideal body weight and create a sense of urgency. Do this by thinking incessantly about your ideal body weight and the benefits associated with its attainment.

When a sense of urgency is developed, you become unstoppable.

By making the attainment of your ideal body weight important to you, giving it value, you assign it urgency. When losing weight is urgent, you are likely to take action.

Embrace change, be enthusiastic about it.
For without change, you are who you are,
not who you could be.

CAUTION

A JOURNEY OF A THOUSAND MILES MUST BEGIN WITH A SINGLE STEP.

Lao-tzu (604-531 B.C.)

CAUTION

USE COMMON SENSE...

The Invisible Diet was NOT constructed to alter your existing day to day activities. Only to facilitate weight loss by doing what you are already doing, and by adding a small component (creating belief by applying autosuggestion).

Therefore, if you are already watching what you eat, exercising regularly, or doing whatever it is you do that is perceived as beneficial, continue doing so.

Do not use ***The Invisible Diet*** as an excuse not to exercise, or act irresponsibly in your consumption of food and beverage.

Also, it is important to follow the recommendations of your physician.

Use common sense. A friend of mine refers to common sense as *uncommon sense*, because so few people have it.

The next section deals with *understanding.* What price do you need to pay for success?

Take responsibility for your actions.

UNDER-
STANDING

IT IS OF ITSELF THAT THE DIVINE THOUGHT THINKS (SINCE IT IS THE MOST EXCELLENT OF THINGS), AND ITS THINKING IS A THINKING ON THINKING.

Aristotle (384-322 B.C.)

UNDERSTANDING

YOU MUST PAY THE PRICE FOR FOR SUCCESS...

It would be a good idea to let you know, right from the start, that all you must do, at specific times of the day, is repeat a special phrase. That is all!

The phrase you are to repeat is simple and precise, and is to be tailored to your expectations.

As a cautionary note, I must say simple repetition of this phrase without a clear understanding of **WHY** you are repeating it, **HOW** you are to repeat it, and **WHEN** you are to repeat it, will most likely result in wasted time and effort.

Think of this book as a puzzle. Each concept/section represents a piece of the puzzle. When you read and comprehend each section, the puzzle pieces fall into place. Your ability to influence your weight increases with the discovery of each new puzzle piece.

Do not make the assumption that just by having this book you will lose weight. A simple perusal is not enough. Read, digest and apply the information for it to be beneficial.

THE INVISIBLE DIET

Do you believe all people who live on golf courses are good golfers? Are people surrounded by books smart? Do not make the assumption that a quick read will solve your weight problem. Read and reread if necessary, so that you may develop a deeper understanding.

This understanding when mixed with action produces tangible results.

The price for success, in this venture, is understanding. Take the time and pay the price. Understand.

Everything happens for a reason.

WHERE DOES THE WEIGHT GO?

ALL PSYCHICAL ACTS WITHOUT EXCEPTION, IF THEY ARE NOT COMPLICATED BY ELEMENTS OF EMOTION...DEVELOP BY WAY OF REFLEX. HENCE, ALL CONSCIOUS MOVEMENTS RESULTING FROM THESE ACTS AND USUALLY DESCRIBED AS VOLUNTARY, ARE REFLEX MOVEMENTS IN THE STRICT SENSE OF THE TERM.

Ivan Mikhailovich Sechenov (1829-1903)

WHERE DOES THE WEIGHT GO?

THE VANISHING ACT...

When you consistently apply ***The Invisible Diet*** excess pounds melt away ever so gradually. There is a law of nature that says, *"For every action there is an opposite reaction*." The **action** here is applying the diet, and the **reaction** is weight loss.

In your case, by inserting the idea of your ideal body weight in your subconscious mind (the action), your subconscious mind prompts you to ask questions of yourself (the reaction).

Do not idly discard these questions!

Keep in mind your ideal body weight and your desire to reach that goal. Believe me, it will be a no brainer decision when the questions occur.

Questions like:

- Should I have a soda today, or water, tea, juice, etc.?
- Could I take the stairs instead of taking the elevator?

- Should I pack a lunch instead or eating out at a fast food place?

You get the idea.

The quality of the questions you ask yourself, coupled with a timely response, determine the extent of your results.

By asking questions, you access an infinite pool of "*ways*" to lose weight. Asking questions of yourself is a powerful tool to assist you in focusing on ways to facilitate weight loss/change.

When you actively address the questions you ask yourself, with this diet in mind, you gradually establish new empowering habits and at the same time chip away at age old habits written in stone.

As your old habits disappear, your new habits emerge. It is during this transition that your weight adjusts accordingly.

Before long, your responses to the questions you ask become automatic and habitual. These responses occur almost without your conscious knowledge, like a reflex, and due to this reason, your weight seems to disappear. At least that will be your perception.

This whole process occurs so naturally that when you do a final weigh in, you will most likely say to yourself: *"How did I lose that weight?* **I did not recall doing anything different!"**

In the old days, a habit was recognized as an article of clothing. Today, a habit is recognized as a consistent behavior we exhibit.

Change your behavior/habit to influence your weight. Create a new wardrobe of habits that fit your perceived new self.

When you are in harmony with your environment, the actions you take at any given moment may seem insignificant. You tend to forget the insignificant actions taken during the day. It is exactly those actions, rather the cumulative effect of these seemingly insignificant actions that lead to your weight loss.

PHASE 2

UNDERSTAND YOUR INNER-SELF AND UNLEASH THE POWER FROM WITHIN

DESIRE

BEHOLDING BEAUTY WITH THE EYE OF THE MIND, HE WILL BE ENABLED TO BRING FORTH, NOT IMAGES OF BEAUTY, BUT REALITIES (FOR HE HAS HOLD NOT OF AN IMAGE BUT OF A REALITY), AND BRINGING FORTH AND NOURISHING TRUE VIRTUE TO BECOME THE FRIEND OF *GOD* AND BE IMMORTAL, IF MORTAL MAN MAY.

Plato (428-348 B.C.)

DESIRE

FUEL FOR THE FIRE...

Desire is similar to a fire. A small fire produces a small amount of heat, or desire. Bonfires create an enormous amount of heat, or desire.

The fuel for your fire (emotion) is the thought of your ideal body weight (desire).

The trick is to turn ordinary desire, your need to lose weight, into an obsession, the bonfire of desire, so that you may effortlessly achieve your ideal body weight.

A crucial step in any weight loss program is recognizing there are numerous degrees of desire. When you understand this concept, you will agree that focusing on ways to elevate your desire enhances your dieting experience.

Turn up the heat, your fire of desire, by becoming more emotional about the achievement of your ideal body weight.

There is a direct linkage between your desire and your emotions. The more you desire your ideal body weight, the more emotional you become.

In other words, the thought of your ideal body weight is impotent when it is not accompanied by favorable emotions.

To intensify the fire of desire, you must mix emotion with your thought. Your emotions act like an arm that throws the fuel on the fire.

Thoughts without feeling/emotion are like a stack of logs sitting next to a fire. They are only potential fuel, and are useful only when added to the fire.

The best way to create beneficial emotions/feelings in you is to see in your minds eye, how you would feel at your ideal body weight, or how it would feel better in your new clothes. Notice in your mind how people would look at you. Notice how you would walk with confidence. Smell the foods you will be eating. Taste the different flavors. Feel your body getting tighter, etc.

The idea here is, during your waking hours, to think of your ideal body weight and visualize yourself at that weight often. This intensifies your emotions with each repetition.

DESIRE

When you create a mental picture of yourself at your ideal body weight, you automatically develop a positive thinking mindset.

By doing this, you become more and more focused on your objective. Efforts that you exert, produce more meaningful results.

Avoid the impulse of desiring to lose weight and feeling you cannot. This produces a mental conflict, that leads to inaction or the achievement of the opposite of what is desired.

Be aware that there is a direct relationship between desire and persistence. The more you desire your ideal body weight, the more likely you are to be persistent in your efforts. Persistence has a way of knocking down all obstacles.

If you find your persistence waning, rekindle the fire of desire, by thinking of the positive ways you will feel when you achieve your ideal weight. See yourself, in your minds eye, at your ideal body weight. Think good thoughts often, this should get you back on track.

A long time ago, the Romans commanded by Julius Caesar invaded what is now called,

Great Britain. At the beginning of the campaign, all of his ships were ordered to be burned so that there would be no retreat. The Roman invaders, being far outnumbered by their adversaries, had two choices, win or perish. They won.

When you instill desire such as this, nothing can stop you from achieving your ideal body weight. There is no such thing as failure when you desire a thing with such intensity.

Burn your ships, watch the smoke drift away, and realize that you must take action now if you are to live a prosperous, healthy and long life.

By leaving no avenue for retreat, you are guaranteeing your ultimate success.

Say to yourself that achieving your ideal body weight is the end all in your life. Then let your congruent actions, thoughts, and words guide you to that final destination.

The following is a lesson in persistence.

Years ago I attended school in a moderate sized mid-western community, and was enrolled in the college of business. While In class, one of my business professors related his knowledge of hiring practices at a local business.

He said that our town had a pharmaceutical that was a prized place of employment because of pay, benefits and the like. It was his understanding that a common employment practice at this institution was the weighing of applicant files. He said that "*once an applicant's file reached a certain weight, that person would be hired. Maybe not for the position they applied for, but for a position all the same.*"

By applying persistence, you are able to achieve similar results.

Establish what it is most important in your life, something you must have or do. Cherish this thought, and accept nothing less than its complete fulfillment.

SUBCONSCIOUS/ CONSCIOUS MIND

WHEN I WAS YOUNGER I COULD REMEMBER ANYTHING, WHETHER IT HAPPENED OR NOT; BUT I AM GETTING OLDER, AND SOON I SHALL REMEMBER ONLY THE LATTER.

(From Albert Bigelow Paine, Mark Twain, a biography 1912)

SUBCONSCIOUS/CONSCIOUS MIND

HOW TO INFLUENCE YOUR SUBCONSCIOUS MIND...

It is my intention to simplify, as much as possible, an extremely complicated subject. You are reading this book to learn how to lose weight the effortless way, not to get a degree in psychology.

Therefore, it is in your best interest to take this stance: **It is not necessary to know completely how something functions to use it.**

For instance, do you need to understand intricately all the inner workings of an automobile to drive somewhere? I really do not think so. Sure, it is good to know how to read the fuel gauge, and how to turn on the lights.

To yield the weight loss you desire, you must understand certain things about the conscious and subconscious mind.

What you need to comprehend is that there is an interaction between the conscious and subconscious mind, and that ***you can influence* that interaction**. Furthermore, you must understand the dynamics of your mind.

THE INVISIBLE DIET

Your mind has two distinct spheres of activity, one conscious and the other subconscious.

The **conscious mind** is objective and voluntary in nature. The conscious mind is your reasoning mind. It helps you make informed decisions, sets goals, etc. Whenever you say to yourself, I want this, or I want that, you are employing the conscious mind. Your desire is a conscious activity. When you go to sleep it rests also.

The **subconscious mind** is subjective and involuntary in nature. It keeps your body running; for instance it keeps your circulatory system functioning, it repairs injuries to the body; it keeps you breathing even when you are asleep. It is the seat of your imagination and is the storehouse of knowledge. Influenced by suggestion, it does what it is told. It does not reason, it accepts what is impressed upon it as truth. It is your true source of **power**. Sleep walking and sleep talking are examples of subconscious expression.

Your subconscious mind rules the roost. It ultimately determines your course of action.

SUBCONSCIOUS/CONSCIOUS MIND

The conscious mind is a weakling in comparison.

Look at it this way; you have a place you need to go to, so you pick up the phone and call a travel agency and speak to a travel agent. Your destination, in this case, is your conscious desire. The travel agent, in this case, is your subconscious mind.

Ask the travel agent to send you to the worst place on Earth, and the travel agent will not argue with you, but simply provide you with a means to get there.

Ask the travel agent to send you to the best place on Earth, and soon you will find yourself there.

Be very specific in your desire; also be careful what you desire.

The subconscious mind, your travel agent, finds a way to speed you to the destination of your choice without judgment. All the agent asks for, in advance, is the fare.

The fare in this case is **belief,** belief that you are entitled to something; belief that you can do something; belief that you are smart enough, etc. When you produce the fare, you get places. Without the fare, you are stuck where you are.

Create a sense of belief that you can lose weight; put your subconscious mind on notice that it has a job to do.

By creating belief in yourself, you are automatically influencing your subconscious mind.

When you claim to desire weight loss and you have not established a sense of belief, then the subconscious mind gives you the opposite of what you desire.

Why? Because your subconscious mind is not getting a clear message, therefore it is unable to help you. Any hint of doubt, exposes your true belief, and it is that belief the subconscious mind acts upon.

Thinking of a combination of good and bad thoughts, during the day, sends mixed messages to your subconscious mind.

SUBCONSCIOUS/CONSCIOUS MIND

The thoughts you entertain must be either all good, or all bad, if they are to send a clear message to your subconscious mind. Believe me, it is definitely in your best interest to think good thoughts.

Bouncing back and forth between good and bad thoughts is similar to telling a travel agent you want to go here, here, here and here -- NOW. The travel agent will think you are crazy and do nothing because the agent has no clear destination. Your subconscious mind will leave you in the lurch when you act similarly.

You must learn to communicate with your subconscious mind in order to lose weight.

During the waking day, the subconscious mind does **not** accept any orders from your conscious mind that have not been colored with belief. In other words, unless you firmly **believe** something to be true, telling yourself otherwise produces the opposite result.

It is your dominating feelings, no matter how great or small that are acted upon by the subconscious mind.

A good example of this is: You want to lose weight, and you say so. But deep inside, you believe/feel that it is a waste of time, etc. Are you likely to lose weight in this scenario? Not likely! It is absurd to believe otherwise.

What you have to do is back your thought with a congruent emotion. Positive thought with positive emotion. When your thoughts and emotions do not match, your subconscious mind accepts only the dominating emotion.

The door to the subconscious mind is always open to your dominating feelings. These feelings are accepted without challenge and are immediately acted upon, because they are something you believe to be true.

The door to the subconscious mind is always closed to thoughts/desires that are not fully believed in.

This is a huge reason why people do not lose weight and keep it off.

Now, the trick is being able to establish a desire, and find a way to slip through the door to your subconscious mind by creating belief that you can lose weight.

SUBCONSCIOUS/CONSCIOUS MIND

Look at it this way. When you need a new key made, you bring the original key to a store. The person at the store finds a "*blank*", a key that can be ground as a duplicate. Then the store clerk places the blank in a key grinding machine. When the process is done, you have a new key that allows you passage where you need to go.

When you have a desire, you must open the door to your subconscious mind with a key. The key is developed this way:

- **Your desire is the "blank" key**
- **Autosuggestion (see BELIEF section) represents the grinding machine**
- **The finished KEY is BELIEF**

No conscious desire is allowed to enter the subconscious mind without the key of belief.

Remember, the whole idea is to convey, to your subconscious mind, the message that you intend to achieve your ideal body weight. Then leave it up to the subconscious mind to lead and guide you to your desired goal.

Another example is in order:

THE INVISIBLE DIET

When you send an e-mail on the computer you must type the message (thought), enter an e-mail address (destination) and finally hit the "*send*" key, otherwise the message is useless.

If you do not get a response, it behooves you to continue sending messages until you get one.

Think of the message as the thought of your ideal body weight, the destination as being your subconscious mind, and the send button as the constant repetition of your desire (autosuggestion).

In the absence of strong desire backed up with belief, your subconscious mind is influenced by the way you feel emotionally, and many people are an emotional mess. Taken a step further, the way you look is a direct result of how you feel.

This is why so many people have weight problems and in life in general, they do not comprehend the relationship between their conscious and subconscious mind.

To be simplistic, your day is composed of:

- Sleep hours
- Awake hours

SUBCONSCIOUS/CONSCIOUS MIND

Hopefully, the majority of your time is awake, so it would be most prudent to follow the above advice.

Now, for sleep!

The easiest and hardest time to send messages to your subconscious mind is just prior to falling asleep, and just after you wake up.

I say it is easy to convey messages to your subconscious mind at this time because your conscious mind is at its weakest at this moment. If you have thoughts that are negative in nature, they disappear. Your subconscious mind penetrates your conscious mind, at this time, and absorbs like a sponge all conscious suggestions.

It is the hardest time to send messages because you must develop discipline to keep from falling asleep and you must convey, in a monotone voice, predetermined messages so as not to stir up emotion. Also, you must make sure to move your lips and be able to hear yourself.

Now you understand there are two times a day that you can influence your subconscious mind through conscious suggestion. Take advantage of that knowledge.

One last thought before you move on.

Think of your subconscious mind as a piece of modeling clay. You are endeavoring to construct an image of you at your ideal body weight. Each positive emotions/feelings provides further definition. When negative emotions/feelings come about, they stamp on the clay figure and flatten it out. No matter how much work you have put into it, you must start anew.

When you have developed conviction, the image is complete and the subconscious mind breathes life into it. At this point your desire develops a magnetic attraction and draws to you all that is necessary for the fulfillment of that desire.

How can you influence your subconscious mind to achieve your dietary goals? Let us examine the establishment of belief.

SUBCONSCIOUS/CONSCIOUS MIND

The subconscious mind can be your friend or your foe. Make it your friend by influencing it, and by making suggestions to it at the proper time of the day, when it is least distracted by your conscious thought.

BELIEF

MEN WILLINGLY BELIEVE WHAT THEY WISH.

Julius Caesar (100-44 B.C.)

BELIEF

CONSTRUCT BELIEF THROUGH AUTOSUGGESTION...

My definition of belief is: accepting something to be true.

For ***The Invisible Diet*** to work for you, belief must be established. Belief that when the diet is applied consistently and persistently it will, with time, produces the results you seek. Belief that the words you speak are **TRUE.**

Convince yourself that you can lose weight, knowing that weight loss is possible, then you are able to do it without regard to its level of difficulty.

Reverse the situation, when you imagine you cannot lose the least amount of weight, you will not.

I look at belief as a bridge that spans from (conscious) desire to (subconscious) imagination. With this bridge you can obtain **any thing** that you desire. Without it, you can obtain **no thing**. You must build the bridge of belief to lose weight.

Let me clarify this.

THE INVISIBLE DIET

Recall the example at the beginning of the book that dealt with walking a mile across a sandy beach during a hurricane? From this example alone, you can clearly see that the subconscious mind makes the ultimate decision whether you will have, achieve, or do anything. You and I daily want **things**, whether we get these things or not is purely dependent upon our beliefs.

Realizing that your ideal body weight is something you greatly desire, you must instill a sense of belief in yourself so that the desired results may be produced.

To establish belief is to build a **mental** bridge. How do you establish belief?

You must repeat a custom made phrase to yourself, and I will soon show you how to do that. That's right; **repeat your phrase over and over again**. The more you repeat that phrase, the more you come to believe in it. It becomes more and more real to you in your imagination and eventually manifests itself in physical expression.

When you repeat something to yourself, emotions well up from within.

BELIEF

Think about it. Do you not become flustered or turn shades of red when you are embarrassed?

Do you not become angry and express that through facial expressions, physical motions and speech when you think repeated thoughts that provoke you in a bad way? This is an outward expression of your feelings. The feelings you dwell upon, think of repeatedly, come to express themselves outwardly.

This accounts for our existing condition. When you repeat something to yourself, you are basically labeling yourself. Now that you have labeled yourself, you must live up to that label or expectation that you have created. Your body responds appropriately to your programming.

When you truly want change in your life, change for the better, you must start by using labels for your benefit.

I am only bringing this up because your quality of life, that of your children's, and all those who come in contact with you, is dependent upon how you feel. Labels influence how you interact with others. Also, how you feel directly affects the way you look.

THE INVISIBLE DIET

Many times the way you feel is influenced by how other people treat you. The interactions between you and others are subject to your labels.

Think about it, when someone says something nice to you, don't you feel good, and is that not reflected by your smiling? Also, if someone says something bad to you, do you not feel disturbed and perhaps frown?

When you deliberately assign positive labels you begin to influence your life, and that of others, for the better.

This goes for the labels you give to the people at work, your husband, your friends and all those you come in contact with.

Once you have created a label, you are compelled to make that label a reality. In other words, you do what you must so as not to disappoint the labeler. So, be careful how you label yourself and others! Create labels that produce positive results; eliminate negative labels.

BELIEF

You can recognize a persons label by just listening to them. When you hear the words *"I am.........*" this is a vocal expression of their label.

Common labels you may hear are, "I am:

- Fat
- Thin
- Healthy
- A clutter bug
- A neat nick
- Stupid
- Smart
- Happy
- Depressed
- Good
- Bad
- A workaholic
- Lazy
- Not a morning person

Listen to yourself when you say: *"I am................"* Take heed, you are labeling.

The problem with people, in most cases, is they did not create the labels they now must live up to. They were initially suggestions from friends, neighbors, family and strangers that they eventually came to accept.

When you were in school, didn't the students, faculty, friends and family say to you that you were smart, or less than smart, and did you not live up to their expectations.

Once you recognize the power labels have on you, just substitute empowering labels for debilitating ones to provide the desired results.

Why not say to yourself:

I am becoming:

- Thin
- Happy
- Healthy
- Active
- Adventurous
- Smarter than I think
- A good person
- Etc.

By taking this approach, you can create lasting change when you come to believe in the power of your labels.

BELIEF

When you repeat something to yourself enough you come to believe in it.

Faith or belief is created when you consciously repeat certain affirmations (your phrase) directed to your subconscious mind. This process is known as ***"AUTOSUGGESTION"*** or self suggestion.

When you repeat your phrase to yourself, you are employing *"autosuggestion."*

The objective here is to influence your subconscious mind so that you may believe that you will achieve your ideal body weight. When you say that you intend to lose weight repeatedly, your subconscious mind comes to accept that suggestion as truth, and expresses that truth as reality.

This suggestion can be true or not, that has little bearing. Have you ever heard of people beating the polygraph test? I believe they are using autosuggestion to achieve their desired result. This also accounts for our remembering things that have never happened.

Your **belief** is constructed by repeating your suggestion until it is accepted by your subconscious mind. The subconscious mind draws you closer to your goals/desires when belief is firmly rooted.

Establish belief in yourself and the diet by doing as follows:

You are to repeat this phrase: **YES, MY IDEAL BODY WEIGHT IS __________ POUNDS. MAKE IT SO BY __________.**

Just fill in the blanks. This is your suggestion.

There are different levels of belief. Take this for example: Think of the person who claims to believe in God, but does not pray or even go to a place of worship. I would say that this person has a superficial level of belief.

Compare that to the individual who proclaims to believe in God. This person prays daily and more than frequents a place of worship. I would say that this person's belief borders on conviction. That is right, **conviction**. Notice how repetition comes into play.

BELIEF

So, you can see from these two examples that there are various degrees of belief.

What you need to do is create conviction in yourself to achieve your ideal body weight.

The level of your belief is reflected by your consistent action. The only real action ***The Invisible Diet*** requires of you is the repetition of your customized phrase and the development of belief that, by repeating this phrase, change for the better must occur.

You can actually see the level of a person's belief by observing their daily actions. This is how one may recognize a person's level of belief, by observing their consistent actions.

Stand back and look at yourself. Are you taking the daily actions necessary to reach your weight loss goal? This should give you some indication of your level of belief in any weight loss program.

Your weight loss results are a direct reflection of the level of belief you have in yourself and the diet, along with the quality and number of actions you take. The actions you end up taking are directly influenced by your beliefs.

THE INVISIBLE DIET

When you create a desire, there is an associated cost. The price you pay is the development of belief. Once you have paid the price, the subconscious mind releases the prize to you.

If you believe you can do a thing,
you will.
If you believe you cannot do a thing,
you won't.
It all comes down to *belief,*
whether you *do* or *don't.*

EMOTIONS

MUCH WATER GOETH BY THE MILL THAT THE MILLER KNOWETH NOT OF.

John Heywood (1497-1580)

EMOTIONS

EMOTIONS LEAD TO MOTION...

Belief requires a solid foundation to rest upon or it disappears from sight. Do not build on quicksand, build on rock.

You must believe in ***The Invisible Diet*** and support it with favorable emotions in order to lose weight.

The foundation of which I am speaking consists of your dominating thoughts/emotions. How you feel, these feelings constitute the message sent to your subconscious mind.

Positive emotions such as: anticipation, expectation, hope and desire provide a foundation of rock.

Expressions like:

- This is easy.
- Today is great.

Negative emotions such as: doubt, anxiety, fear and indecision lay a foundation of sand.

THE INVISIBLE DIET

Expressions like:

- This is difficult.
- I am not sure if I can do this.

Choose to build a sound foundation for belief by expressing yourself in a positive manner.

The words you speak, influence the way you feel, it is simple as that.

A good thing to understand about emotions is that you can entertain only one emotion at a time. **You do not feel good and bad at the same time. You either feel good, or you feel bad.** By recognizing this fact you can, at any time, make yourself feel good by replacing your current negative thought with a pleasant or good one.

Why feel bad, when you can feel good?

Unbridled emotions are much like a sailboat without a rudder. Hop on board, and you end up "*who knows where.*"

Now, reverse the situation. Put a rudder on the sailboat, and then jump on. You are more likely to get to a place of your choosing. Guess who is in control now? This only happens when you keep your emotions in check.

Understanding this fact about emotions, you must respond swiftly when confronted with negative emotions.

It seems that you are most susceptible to negative emotions when you have nothing to do. So, one of the easiest ways to keep negative emotions at bay is to keep busy.

Just think about it, when you are driving home after a long days work and you have no particular thing in mind, don't you become annoyed at other peoples actions (courtesy) or lack thereof on the highway? Isn't it easy to lose your temper? Have you ever witnessed otherwise sane people doing idiotic things?

You must realize that you are being held captive by negative emotions because you are not engaged in productive thought.

When you are most free, and are supposed to be your happiest, is when you are most tormented by negative, debilitating thought. At this time, the smallest observation of something negative is magnified. Is it not ironic that this free time that you cherish most comes at such a high price?

The cruise ship operators know this well. They provide seemingly endless entertainment opportunities to keep you busy so that you have no time to think negative thoughts.

The easiest way to prevent a mutiny on a navy vessel of old was to keep its crew busy. Keep your mind busy, otherwise suffer the consequences of negative thought.

A quick way to snap out of a negative state of mind, or feel better emotionally, is first, to recognize that you have a problem. Then use your body to bring about emotional change, by straightening your back, holding your head high and breathing deep breaths. By doing this, you automatically feel better. You are using physiology to achieve a pleasant feeling.

Use autosuggestion to rid yourself of negative thoughts/emotions. This is how.

As soon as you recognize a negative thought,

counter it with a repeated positive question. By doing this, you shift your attention to a solution, rather than dwell upon the problem.

Questions like:

- How can I make this better?
- How can I get this done faster?
- How can I make my wife feel better?
- What can I do to make our house a happier place?
- How can I lose weight faster?

When repeated to yourself, produce positive results in your life.

Questions like:

- Why does this always happen to me?
- Why do I always feel so bad?
- Why don't my children, husband, wife, boss etc. appreciate me?
- Why can't I lose any weight?

When repeated to yourself, produce negative results in your life.

How you feel at any moment is primarily determined by the *"questions"* you ask yourself.

THE INVISIBLE DIET

When you ask yourself a question, you are shifting your focus. You are looking for answers to your questions. By doing this, you certainly find plenty of answers, both negative and positive, depending upon your focus.

Have you ever listened to a group of individuals gossiping about a certain person? When one person chimes in with a positive comment, further positives are offered. That goes for negative comments also, expose one and an avalanche of negativity is sure to follow.

Negative emotions are the flies at the picnic that land on your food. They seem to come from nowhere and everywhere. They simply appear out of the blue. It is your responsibility to keep the flies away from your food or desire. To do this, you must be vigilant, recognize the problem, and act quickly.

Touch boiling water for a fraction of a second causes no harm. Keep in contact with it for much longer and you experience pain. That goes for negative emotions also. Do not let them take safe harbor in you.

EMOTIONS

Think of negative emotions as being termites that are encroaching on your beautiful wood home. You must, and will do all that is necessary to keep the deadly pests at bay. If you do not recognize the problem, then all is lost.

People receive vaccinations to prevent illness. To prevent the negative emotions (a form of subconscious illness) from welling up in you, I suggest the following.

In the event you are determined to conquer, or at least influence your emotions and make them work for you, read a section called **THE SEVEN DAY MENTAL DIET** in Emmet Fox's book called **POWER THROUGH CONSTRUCTIVE THINKING.**

This short section, when understood and applied, will work miracles for you.

Cleanse yourself of negative thoughts and emotions. Negative thoughts are like a dirty window dividing you from belief. Wipe the window clean with positive thoughts so that you may observe belief.

PHASE 3

LOOK AT THINGS A LITTLE DIFFERENTLY AND APPLY YOUR KNOWLEDGE

TIME

WISELY AND SLOW; THEY STUMBLE THAT RUN FAST.

William Shakespeare

TIME

MAKE TIME YOUR FRIEND...

Work in three month intervals. Then, once you have mastered this program, alter the time span to fit your needs. By doing this you set a **deadline**.

It is my understanding the word "*deadline*" was coined during the American Civil War. Certain prisoner of war camps, due to the lack of building materials, were constructed without walls. Instead, the prison guards drew a line on the ground and told the prisoners that anyone who crossed the line would be killed. The line soon became known as the "*deadline*."

What you are going to do is establish a deadline so that you may realize your ideal body weight. This puts pressure on you.

Deadlines are most effective when coupled with stiff penalties for inaction or failure.

Today, the utilization of deadlines spurs people to action. A classic example is April $15^{th.}$ Our government compels us to act by a specific date regarding tax filing. If you choose not to file, or file late, there are penalties.

There are other dates that come to mind where penalties can be stiff if you forget or ignore them:

- Birthdays
- Anniversaries
- Fathers day
- Mothers day
- Christmas
- Valentine's day
- Etc., etc., etc.

Whether you do a thing or not depends on how important it is to you. That is referred to as a value. When you value something, it is important to you.

If I were to miss a significant event or date, I would never hear the end of it. That is good enough to get me moving.

The easiest way to make a new friend is to find a way to make that person feel important. The easiest way to lose weight is to make ***The Invisible Diet*** your friend by making it important.

Sometimes a value is created when a person *expects* something of you. If you desire to please that person, you must value and assign importance to the things that person finds important. Then you think alike. As they say, "*you are on the same page*." This is a great way to eliminate conflict in relationships.

Create a value, one that you cannot accept anything less than your ideal body weight by a certain date. Make it simply unacceptable to achieve anything less than your ideal body weigh by that time.

Now, let's get back to why setting three month increments is preferable.

Three months sounds like a long time to wait for your initial results. It really is not. This is simply your first perception.

There is an old saying, "*Rome was not built in a day.*" Be patient allowing ample time for your subconscious mind to accept, as belief, your repeated suggestion.

Remember, the whole idea of losing weight is not to see the numbers; it is to feel and look better.

Do not let the idea of three months hinder you. As time progresses, you experience subtle changes in yourself. You feel better, your clothes fit more comfortably, life has more purpose, etc. This should be reinforcement enough.

If this diet is important for you, you will find the time to apply it. I believe that time expands to fit your NEEDS (deepest desires), not your WANTS (superficial desires). In other words, you always can find plenty of time to accomplish what MUST be done.

The Invisible Diet grows on you when given a chance, and before long you look forward to applying it.

Time goes by either quickly or slowly depending on your perspective. If you do not look forward to something the time goes slowly. When you look forward to something, time passes quickly.

There is a fellow who came up with a name for the above phenomenon; he called it **Zeno's Paradox,** which basically says that a unit of time like a minute, can be broken down into infinitesimal smaller units and this can go on forever.

This accounts for the sensation of something taking forever to accomplish.

When you put your mind fully on the task at hand, rather than where you would rather be, time seems to go by quickly and the task becomes effortless.

Have you ever noticed that most successful people enjoy what they are doing? Learn from them. Enjoy applying this diet and you become successful.

Keep focused on ***The Invisible Diet*** and time will be your friend.

Time passes like the waters of a great river. We can stand there and look at the spectacle or immerse ourselves in it. By committing to a plan, establishing consequences, and taking action, we jump into the river and are swept into success, while others are left behind.

TARGET WEIGHT

**LOVE OUR PRINCIPLE,
ORDER OUR FOUNDATION,
PROGRESS OUR GOAL.**

Auguste Comte (1798-1857)

TARGET WEIGHT

Setting goals...

The further away you set a target\goal the less likely you are to hit the mark, and that goes for setting an ideal target weight.

Take for example basketball: If I were to give you a basketball and say, "*Make this basket and I will give you $5,000.*" But you are 200 feet away from the goal! You will automatically say to yourself, "*this is unbelievable*", and you will not put across any serious effort.

Furthermore, I would be willing to bet that you would not even attempt the shot if the $5,000 was to come out of your pocket if you missed the shot.

Now, reverse the situation. You are twelve feet from the basket. Your confidence level increases because you are much closer to your goal. Therefore you are likely to attempt the shot (take action).

By moving an unrealistic goal closer, you increase your level of confidence that the goal/desire is achievable.

Get the idea? Move your target weight (ideal body weight) closer to you in order to make it more believable. By doing this, you increase confidence in yourself, which fosters persistence and **belief.**

You do not run a marathon without training for it. By starting off slowly, just a few miles a day, you are able to gradually increase your endurance, and your belief, to the point where you are able to complete the race that you trained for. This concept should work well with dieting also. Just start slowly.

With your diet experience, create a sense of adventure and let each new experience bring you closer to a happier and more fulfilling life.

So, now you understand that making something appear believable, and coupling that believability, with a strong desire, leads to the development of persistence.

The task here is not to make the target weight too easy or too hard to achieve.

When you set a believable target weight, you

are more likely to be persistent in your efforts. You might say that by setting more difficult goals you are introducing the doubt factor. Mr. Doubt grows larger and larger when you set unrealistic goals.

Your target weight does not have to be your final ideal body weight. It can be simply a way to step down to your ideal body weight. In other words, this can be a temporary goal.

Imagine you are at the top of a flight of stairs. It would be in your best interest to take the steps down one at a time gradually, not racing down them for safety's sake.

By utilizing this concept, you are gradually getting closer and closer to your target weight.

Two things happen when you set a goal.

- You identify an objective.
- You align your focus and magnify it.

Your goal here is to identify your ideal body weight. In other words, figure out what weight you intend to achieve.

THE INVISIBLE DIET

Establish in your mind an exact weight you *must* achieve. Do not confuse this with how much weight you want to lose, for example, ten pounds.

The above statement is of critical importance.

Now that you are focused on your final desired weight, your mind is on constant vigil to find ways to achieve that weight.

Otherwise, when you focus on how much weight you want to lose (your overweight condition), your mind seeks to please you by finding ways to justify it.

Just like a person asked by their boss to reveal all that is good about a product, that person is compelled to search high and low to find something good to say.

In the case of the person asked to tell all that is bad about a product, that person responds appropriately by diligently searching for something bad to say.

Focus clearly on your ideal body weight, your mind searches diligently for ways to reach your objective.

TARGET WEIGHT

Let's get to the nuts and bolts of setting your goal.

Determine, by any means you please, your desired ideal body weight. **MAKE IT BELIEVABLE.**

- Weigh yourself to determine your current weight.
- Subtract your current weight from your ideal weight.
- If you are anywhere from one to fifteen pounds overweight, one three month span should do the trick.
- Anything over fifteen pounds overweight requires further time and effort.

For instance, if you are thirty pounds overweight it may take six months to correct. To lose forty-five pounds, it could take nine months. You get the idea.

After you have achieved positive results, your belief becomes stronger in the system and in yourself; therefore you should be able to set progressively more challenging goals. All you need to do is adjust the figures you place in the above table to reflect your new expectations.

Be careful when initially setting your goal.

With time and persistence you should be able to produce more extraordinary results.

These are the primary elements for establishing your target weight/ideal body weight:

- Use any means you please to figure what weight you desire.
- Make the goal believable.
- Make the goal challenging.
- Increase your expectation with time and favorable experience.

If you do not know where you want to go, how can you ever get there...

THE SCALE

TAKE THEREFORE NO THOUGHT FOR THE MORROW: FOR THE MORROW SHALL TAKE THOUGHT FOR THE THINGS OF ITSELF. SUFFICIENT UNTO THE DAY IS THE EVIL THEREOF.

(Bible. Matthew Ch. VI, V. 34)

THE SCALE

AN EXERCISE IN SELF CONTROL...

I believe many people use the scale to determine how they should feel on any given day. They look to it for advice, as if it were some mystical oracle, so that they may feel justified in their thoughts and actions.

Scales are not designed for that purpose. They are designed to provide information, and in your case a specific body weight.

It is how you interpret that information that determines your course of action, not how you should feel.

Picture this: You encounter a large pile of laundry that you know must be done, and done by you. When you discover this pile unexpectedly, you do not stand there saying to yourself:

- This is the end of the world!
- This is the worst day of my life!
- I cannot believe this!
- Someone shoot me!

NO. NO. NO

THE INVISIBLE DIET

You observe the problem and take immediate action; otherwise the problem only gets worse with time.

The same goes for your body weight and the emotions that lead to your current condition.

After weighing yourself, do not say:

- I am a bad person!
- There is nothing I can do!
- Losing weight is impossible!
- I am resigned to this weight!

NO. NO. NO.

Get a grip on the situation.

When the weight, as reflected by the scale, does not match your expectation, reflect on your ideal body weight and control your emotions.

Weigh yourself at a prescribed time that you set in your plan. By keeping away from the scale, until then, your focus should be on your ideal weight, not your existing weight.

THE SCALE

Accept the information conveyed to you as being helpful, whether you like it or not. Then take corrective measures when necessary.

PLAN

NOT SNOW, NO, NOR RAIN, NOR HEAT, NOR NIGHT KEEPS THEM FROM ACCOMPLISHING THEIR APPOINTED COURSES WITH ALL SPEED.

Herodotus (485-425 B.C.)

PLAN

A COURSE OF ACTION...

Actually, a plan to me is nothing more than a map with a highlighted route to your destination. The highlighted route being the actions, or sequence of actions, you must take consistently to reach your ideal body weight destination.

The development of this plan is easy.

Let me show you how.

<u>**STEP # 1**</u>

This is the plan. You are to repeat this phrase: **"Yes, my ideal body weight is _________ pounds. Make it so by ____________."**

Just fill in the gaps and make it believable.

<u>**STEP #2**</u>

Now, you must repeat your custom phrase twenty times before you go to sleep at night, and twenty times just after you wake in the morning while in bed.

This sounds easy until you try it. Like lifting exercise weights, your thoughts at that moment are heavy and require effort to express verbally. With time and repetition, this becomes easier.

To ensure persistence, before you jump into bed and just prior to getting out of bed, think of how good it will feel when you reach your goal.

Repeat the phrase while lying in bed with your eyes closed, moving your lips so that you can hear yourself. You can do this in a low tone so as not to disturb others. Remember, do this twenty times.

When you repeat the phrase, make sure not to think of anything in particular. Just say the phrase in a **monotonous** tone. Do not invoke emotion.

At this point you should be in, what is recognized as, a meditative state, and in this state, your suggestions should be well received by the subconscious mind.

You are basically sculpting the subconscious mind just like a body builder would do except your exercise is purely mental.

PLAN

STEP #3

On the date you have decided to reach your ideal body weight, you will weigh yourself.

STEP #4

When you reach your desired weight you can maintain it by repeating to yourself: "**My ideal body weight is _________.**"

From this point on, all you need to do is recite this custom phrase to yourself at the appropriate times in the prescribed way.

STEP #5

In the event, you did not reach your desired weight; go to the problem solving section of the book. You have to make adjustments.

A word of caution; Keep what you are doing to yourself until positive meaningful results are achieved. Otherwise, you may be swayed by the opinion of others.

I once heard a person say: "*Ninety percent of the people we encounter could care less about our problems, five percent are concerned about us and our problems, and the remaining five percent are glad we have them."*

Thorough plans dispel doubt and foster belief.

PROBLEM SOLVING

KNOWLEDGE MUST COME THROUGH ACTION; YOU CAN HAVE NO TEST WHICH IS NOT FANCIFUL, SAVE BY TRIAL.

Sophocles (495-406 B.C.)

PROBLEM SOLVING

LET'S GET THIS RIGHT...

In the event you did not achieve your ideal body weight or temporary goal by the allotted day, take note.

When you apply ***The Invisible Diet,*** please understand this concept: **There is no such thing as wrong or right or anything in between, only results.**

Do not confuse the above concept for giving yourself permission to act irresponsibly. You already know right from wrong. What I am really trying to say is this: People learn from their mistakes. Make many mistakes, and you should learn plenty.

My experience is that people who are more successful than I am have simply made more mistakes than I have.

An example is in order: When a pilot flies a plane to any destination, the pilot must make course adjustments to keep on track. Winds, weather and the like can cause the plane to veer off course. When the pilot recognizes the plane is off course, the pilot takes immediate corrective measures. The pilot, in this case is neither right, nor wrong, only adjusting to the current condition to achieve the desired result.

Do not get all worked up about whether you were right or wrong. Simply take corrective action.

The corrective action, you most likely have to take, is to reread this book, or certain sections, to get a deeper understanding of the principles involved. How hard can that be?

Evaluate the situation. How much weight did you lose? Did you lose any weight?

Then figure:

- ❖ Did you establish a believable ideal body weight?
- ❖ Did you provide enough time for the process?
- ❖ Were the steps to reaching your ideal body weight compatible/believable?

The best laid plans do not work if they are not **believable**. Eliminate all doubt in your mind by rereading this book or sections that you find important. By reading something repeatedly, you come to believe in it.

Next, did you repeat your custom phrase twenty times while you were in bed, with your eyes closed?

Did you repeat the phrase by moving your lips and speaking loud enough to hear the words?

You must repeat the phrase in a **monotonous** way making sure not to invoke/ bring about any emotion! The whole idea is to make a suggestion to your subconscious mind, not to tell it what to think or do.

Remember, your subconscious mind is most susceptible to suggestion just prior to falling asleep at night, and just after you wake in the morning.

By repeating, in a monotonous way, you are inscribing in your subconscious mind your intentions without stirring up emotions.

Reading and rereading this book provides you with a deeper understanding of the principles involved. You are employing what the Japanese call "*kaizen*" which means –continual improvement.

When you are given a test once, you either pass or fail it. When you are allowed to study the test and take it repeatedly after analyzing your shortcomings, you are sure to improve.

Rereading this book can only help you.

Renew your persistence. Employ the principles at hand, and success is yours.

Recognize your deficiency, seek counsel, and then take appropriate action.

Made in the USA
Monee, IL
05 November 2026

67969832R10083